THE

ART OF

SHAVING

SHAVING
MADE EASY

What the Man Who
Shaves
Ought to Know

ILLUSTRATED

PUBLISHED BY
THE 20th CENTURY
CORRESPONDENCE SCHOOL
NEW YORK

THIS BOOK
IS DEDICATED TO THOSE
MEN WHO HAVE DIFFICULTIES IN
SHAVING, IN HOPE THAT ITS CONTENTS
WILL BE OF ASSISTANCE IN REMEDYING
THEIR TROUBLES.

v

PUBLISHER'S PREFACE

Let me set the stage for you. It's the early 20th century, and men across the world are shaving with straight razors—tools built to last a lifetime, tools that required skill and care. If they were so good, why doesn't every man still shave with a straight razor? Well, along comes King Gillette, a man with an eye for opportunity and a knack for reshaping the market. He didn't just sell razors; he sold an idea, a revolution, as he liked to call it. But revolutions come with costs, and not all are paid in money. Some cost us more.

What Gillette did was genius, but not the kind of genius that builds monuments or writes symphonies. His was a cold, calculated genius. He looked at the straight razor and saw not an instrument of skill and pride, but a problem: it was too good, too lasting, too self-reliant. You could buy one razor and shave for decades, with nothing more than a bit of soap and a strop. Where's the profit in that?

The Razor-and-Blade Trap

So Gillette turned the world on its head. His business model, now known as the "razor-and-blade" strategy, was devilishly simple. Sell the razor cheaply, sometimes even at a loss, and hook the customer into buying replacement blades for the rest of their life. A renewable revenue stream. The genius wasn't in the product; it was in the cycle.

You see, the safety razor wasn't really about giving you a better shave. It was about making you dependent. You'd never just buy a razor again— you'd buy the razor, then the blades, over and over. Gillette didn't want you to own a tool; he wanted you to own a problem that only his company could solve.

And he succeeded. Oh, how he succeeded. His razors were in every home, his name on every bathroom sink. But the cost of that success wasn't borne by him alone.

The Shaving Skill Set, Lost

Before Gillette, a man's morning shave was more than a routine—it was a ritual. It took patience, care, and no small amount of skill. You had to know your tools, respect them, maintain them. A straight razor was a thing of precision, a blade that demanded your attention. It was unforgiving, yes, but in the best way—it kept you sharp, literally and figuratively.

Gillette sold a shortcut. He sold ease at the expense of mastery. Why bother with the careful art of stropping and honing when you could just swap out a blade? Why take the time to learn a craft when you could let a new piece of disposable steel do the work for you? He didn't just sell convenience; he sold a future where skill and patience were no longer required.

And men bought it. By the millions, they bought it. Over time, the art of shaving with a straight razor—the pride of doing it right, of mastering the blade—faded into obscurity.

A Legacy of Waste

Now let's talk about the environmental cost. Gillette didn't just make shaving easier; he made it wasteful. Those disposable blades, those plastic cartridges—they don't vanish once you've tossed them in the bin. They pile up. Landfills, oceans, wherever we humans tend to dump our refuse. Billions of them, year after year, accumulating like a slow tide of sharp, gleaming detritus.

And for what? For convenience? For a slightly quicker shave? The straight razor, by contrast, is a model of sustainability. One blade, cared for properly, can last a lifetime. No waste, no endless supply chain of blades and plastic handles. But that doesn't make money, does it? Not for the likes of Gillette.

His model helped birth the throwaway culture we're drowning in today. He turned a simple daily act into a cycle of consumption that feeds on itself. A cycle that never ends, unless you decide to break free.

The Illusion of Savings

Here's the kicker: Gillette sold his safety razors as an affordable option. Cheap razors, cheap blades—what's not to love? But those blades add up. Slowly, stealthily, the cost piles on, year after year. By the time you've finished counting, you've spent far more than you would have on a high-quality straight razor and its maintenance.

It's the genius of small increments. You never notice how much you're paying because it comes in drips and drabs. A few dollars here, a few more there. But in the end, you're in for much more than you ever realized. And Gillette knew that. He counted on it.

The Price of Dependency

What Gillette really sold was dependence. He made men reliant on a product that they couldn't maintain or improve on their own. With a straight razor, you control everything—sharpness, technique, the whole process. With a safety razor, you're at the mercy of the next blade pack, the next design tweak, the next price hike.

You become a customer for life, not because you want to be, but because you have no choice. You're locked in. And that, my friend, is the brilliance and the tragedy of Gillette's model. It took something simple and self-sufficient and turned it into a permanent expense.

A Culture of Disposability

Gillette's razor wasn't just a product; it was a symbol. A symbol of the disposable age. His business model helped set the stage for a world where everything is temporary, replaceable, forgettable. We've applied his logic to everything: from coffee pods to smartphones, we've built a society on the idea that nothing should last.

But ask yourself this: is that progress? Or is it just a more elegant form of waste?

Reclaiming the Lost Art

The good news is, it doesn't have to be this way. More and more men are rediscovering the straight razor, reclaiming a skill that should never have been lost. They're stepping out of Gillette's endless cycle and into a world where shaving is more than just a chore. It's a ritual, a craft, a connection to the past.

When you shave with a straight razor, you're doing more than cutting hair. You're making a statement. You're saying that some things are worth doing the right way, not the easy way. You're saying that skill, patience, and sustainability still matter.

Closing Thoughts

So, what do we make of King Gillette? He was a visionary, no doubt. He saw a way to turn a necessity into an empire. But his legacy isn't just about razors and blades. It's about what happens when convenience becomes the ultimate goal, when profit takes precedence over craftsmanship and sustainability.

Gillette changed the game, but it's time we stopped playing by his rules. The straight razor is more than a relic— it's a reminder. A reminder that sometimes, the old ways are better, that skill and self-reliance are worth preserving. So pick up a straight razor. Learn its ways. And carve out a future that respects the past.

EDITOR'S INTRODUCTION

Well now, you've gone and picked up this little book, haven't you? That tells me you're curious, maybe even serious, about learning the old art of straight razor shaving. Good. I'm glad. Pull up a chair, because I'm going to talk to you as I would my own grandson, sharing a bit of wisdom about why this old way of shaving might just be one of the best decisions you'll ever make.

You see, we live in times where everything is fast, disposable, and often more complicated than it needs to be. But sometimes, the old ways turn out to be the best ways. Shaving with a straight razor, the so-called "cut-throat," isn't just a nod to history—it's a practical, satisfying, and downright enjoyable part of a man's life. And let me tell you why.

Escape the Wasteful Modern Razor Game

Let's talk about waste for a moment. You see, those modern razors with their replaceable cartridges and disposable handles might seem convenient, but they're part of a much bigger problem. Every single one of those plastic bits ends up in a landfill or worse, the ocean. They don't decompose, and they won't break down in our lifetimes—or even in our great-grandchildren's lifetimes.

Think about it: billions of these things are discarded every year. It's a staggering number. And for what? A shave that's usually subpar, with blades that dull faster than a pocketknife used on a camping trip. It's an expensive and wasteful cycle, one that most folks never even think twice about.

Now, let's take a moment to reflect on what that means. When you toss out a cartridge razor, you're throwing away more than just plastic and metal. You're discarding the resources and energy it took to produce it, the transportation to get it into your hands, and the waste management to deal with it afterward. Multiply that by millions of men around the world, and you begin to see the scale of the problem.

But you, my friend, are here, and that tells me you're looking for a better way. A straight razor doesn't just save you from contributing to that mountain of plastic waste—it's a stand against the throwaway culture that's taken hold of our world. With a straight razor, you're choosing something permanent, something that you can pass down if you take care of it. A tool that respects the planet and respects you.

Save Your Hard-Earned Money

Now, I know money talks, and here's something you'll want to hear: shaving with a straight razor will save you a tidy sum over the years. Let's break it down.

How many times do you head to the store or order online for more cartridges? Each pack costs a pretty penny, and that's not even counting the fancy cans of shaving foam you pick up alongside them. Over the course of a year, that adds up fast. And then, of course, you've got to replace the handle every so often, because they're not made to last.

Let's do some quick math. Say you're spending $30 every couple of months on cartridges and another $10 or so on shaving cream. That's easily $200 a year, maybe more. Multiply that over a decade, and you're looking at a couple of grand spent on a subpar shave. Now imagine what else you could do with that money.

Compare that to a straight razor. You buy one—just one—and it's yours for life. Sure, you'll need a strop to keep it sharp, and a hone for occasional maintenance, but those aren't recurring expenses. And as for shaving soap, it lasts so much longer than those aerosol cans that it's hardly a comparison. You'll find yourself saving money after just a couple of years, and from then on, it's all profit.

It's an investment, plain and simple. One that pays off not just in the short term but for decades. And the best part? You're getting a superior shave without the constant expense. It's the kind of financial sense that makes you wonder why more people haven't already made the switch.

Mastering a Timeless Skill

There's a bit of magic in learning to use a straight razor. It's not like those multi-blade monstrosities where you can swipe at your face without a second thought. No, this requires precision, patience, and a steady hand. It's a skill, plain and simple, and one that's been passed down for generations.

You'll start slow, of course, and that's part of the beauty. You'll learn the feel of the blade, the right angle to hold it, and the best way to glide it across your face. It'll take a bit of time, and yes, you might nick yourself once or twice. But let me tell you, there's a real satisfaction in mastering something that requires effort and care.

This isn't just about getting a shave—it's about building confidence. Every time you pick up that razor, you're reminding yourself that you've got the skill and the patience to do things right. It's a confidence that carries over into other parts of life, too. After all, if you can master a straight razor, what else might you be capable of?

Learning to shave this way also connects you to something larger. You're not just shaving; you're participating in a craft that has stood the test of time. There's a sense of continuity in that, a feeling that you're part of a long line of men who've honed their blades and their skills. And let me tell you, that's a good feeling.

The Closest, Smoothest Shave

Let's not forget why you're here in the first place: to get the best shave possible. And let me tell you, nothing beats a straight razor. Those modern razors with their rows of blades might promise a close shave, but they often fall short. They tug at your whiskers, irritate your skin, and leave you with razor burn and ingrown hairs.

A straight razor is different. It cuts cleanly and precisely, right at the surface. With the proper technique, you'll get a shave so close your skin will feel like it's never seen a whisker. And because it's just one sharp blade, there's far less irritation. No more red bumps, no more discomfort—just smooth, healthy skin.

This kind of shave isn't just about looks, either. It's about feeling good. When you run your hand over your face after a straight razor shave, you'll know you've done something right. It's a small victory to start your day, and it sets the tone for everything that follows.

But here's the real secret: the more you use a straight razor, the better your shaves will get. Your technique will improve, your skin will adapt, and before long, you'll wonder how you ever settled for anything less.

A Ritual Worth Savoring

Here's where we get into the heart of the matter. Straight razor shaving isn't just about getting the job done— it's about the experience. In our fast-paced world, it's easy to lose sight of the small rituals that make life rich and meaningful. Shaving with a straight razor brings that back.

Think about it: you start by stropping your blade, preparing it for the task ahead. Then there's the lather, made fresh with a brush and a good soap. You take your time, building it up until it's just right. And then, with deliberate care, you shave. Each stroke is measured, each movement purposeful.

This ritual demands your attention. It forces you to slow down and be present in the moment. And in doing so, it turns an ordinary task into something extraordinary. It's a time for reflection, a chance to gather your thoughts and prepare for the day. It's a gift you give yourself every morning, and it's one of the most satisfying parts of the straight razor experience.

There's something grounding about the whole process. It's a reminder that life isn't just about rushing from one task to the next—it's about taking the time to do things well. And in a world that often feels chaotic and hurried, that's a lesson worth remembering.

A Connection to the Past

When you use a straight razor, you're joining a tradition that stretches back through the ages. This isn't just a tool—it's a piece of history. Your great-grandfather might have used one, and his father before him. They knew the value of a good shave, and they understood that some things are worth doing the right way.

There's a certain pride that comes with carrying on that tradition. You're not just shaving—you're honoring the men who came before you. You're keeping alive a skill that's stood the test of time, and you're passing it on to the next generation. It's a way of connecting with your roots, with the craftsmanship and wisdom of those who paved the way.

And here's the thing: this isn't just about looking back. It's about bringing the past into the present, about finding value in traditions that still have so much to offer. In a world that often prizes the new over the tried-and-true, that's a powerful statement.

A Step Towards Self-Reliance

In a world where we're so often dependent on technology and disposable products, straight razor shaving is a refreshing act of self-reliance. You don't need a drawer full of replacement blades or a monthly subscription to keep you going. All you need is your razor, your strop, and a bit of skill.

It's a simple setup, but it gives you everything you need. And in a way, it's a reminder that you're capable of more than you might think. You're taking care of yourself, with your own hands and your own tools. There's a quiet strength in that, and it's something to be proud of.

Self-reliance isn't just about shaving, of course. It's a mindset, a way of approaching the world. It's about taking responsibility for your own needs and finding satisfaction in the things you can do for yourself. And in a time when so much is outsourced or automated, that's a rare and valuable thing.

Ready to Begin?

So here you are, holding the very guide that'll help you get started. This little book has all the knowledge you need to take your first steps into the world of straight razor shaving. It'll teach you how to choose a razor, care for it, and master the technique.

You might feel a bit nervous at first—that's natural. But remember, every master was once a beginner.

Take your time, follow the advice here, and before long, you'll wonder how you ever shaved any other way.

Welcome to a tradition that's as rewarding as it is practical. I'm glad you're here. Now, let's get you started on a journey that'll last a lifetime.

ORIGINAL 1905 PREFACE.

The object of this little book is to furnish clear and full information about the art of shaving. There are few men who do not experience more or less difficulty in shaving themselves, and many who, after a few unsuccessful attempts, give it up in despair and go to the barber shop. We believe most of these would much prefer to shave themselves if only they could do as well as a barber.

The advantages, indeed, seem to be wholly with the man who shaves himself. In the first place the shaving is done in the privacy of his own room. He has his own razor, cup, soap, brush and towels, which can be kept scrupulously clean and sanitary, thus avoiding the constant danger of infection. There is no long wait for the call of "next." After the first cost of the outfit there is nothing to pay, either for services or "tips." Thus in point of time, money and health, the man who shaves himself is a decided gainer.

There are few things in life that are really difficult to perform when one thoroughly knows how to do them. Shaving is no exception. The art of shaving can be easily acquired if one only has the will, and the necessary practical information. This book, which, as far as we are aware, is the only one treating the subject at all completely, endeavors to supply such information; as well for the improvement of men accustomed to shave themselves, as for the instruction of beginners. We believe that any man who will carefully read and follow the instructions here given, will, with some little practice, soon be able to shave himself easily and even better than the barber can do it for him.

CONTENTS.

The Art of Shaving:
Shaving Made Easy
What the Man Who Shaves
Ought to Know

I.
THE SHAVING OUTFIT.

First-class tools are necessary at the very outset. No matter how skillfully one may handle inferior tools, they will invariably produce poor results.

Probably as many failures have resulted from the use of poor razors, strops, or soap as from the lack of knowledge how to use them. In order that the best possible results may be attained, good tools and skill in using them should go hand in hand.

The shaving outfit should consist of one or two good razors, a first-class strop, a mirror, a cup, a brush, a cake of shaving soap, and a bottle of either bay rum, witch hazel, or some other good face lotion. These constitute what may be considered the necessary articles, and to these may be added a number of others, such as a good hone, magnesia or talcum powder, astringent or styptic pencils, antiseptic lotions, etc. which, while not absolutely requisite, will nevertheless add much to the convenience, comfort and luxury of the shave.

II.
THE RAZOR.

The most important article of the shaving outfit is of course the razor, and upon its selection your success or failure in self-shaving will largely depend. Never purchase a razor because it happens to be cheap; a poor razor is dear at any price. You want not the cheapest, but the best.

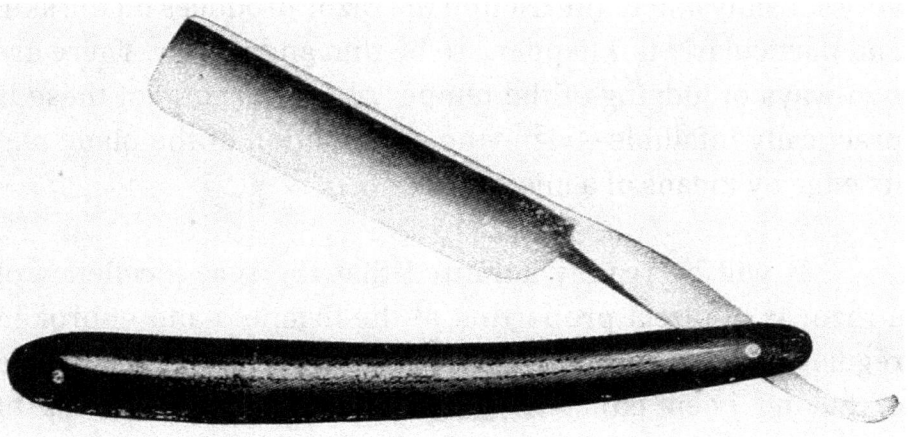

AN IDEAL RAZOR.

A *good* razor if rightly used, will last for years, and will be a source of continual pleasure when used, whereas a *poor* razor will do inferior work, irritate the skin and make the face sore, and be a continual source of trouble and annoyance. If you have such a razor, the sooner you throw it aside and substitute a good one, the better.

The principal point to be considered in selecting a razor is the quality of the steel. By "quality" is meant its *temper* or degree of solidity, and its consequent capability of receiving, even after a series of years, a firm and fine edge. This is undoubtedly the first point to which the purchaser should give attention. By what means though, can he judge of the temper of a razor without using it? The unassisted eye is not sufficient. Its power extends no further than to the discovery of defects the most striking and injurious. The irregularities in a razor's edge, which arise from improper tempering and lack of skill in working, are usually so minute, that they may remain undistinguished until the razor is used. They will nevertheless very sensibly add to the friction the razor produces on the skin and particularly if it happens to be thin and tender. There are two ways of judging of the temper of a razor; one of these is practically infallible—viz:—the examination of the blade and its edge by means of a microscope.

It will be readily admitted that the real excellence of a razor is in direct proportion to the firmness and unbroken regularity of its edge. When a razor is too brittle, in consequence of having been either to much heated in the process of hardening, or not sufficiently cooled in that of tempering, it cannot possibly take a good cutting edge, no matter how much skill may be employed in honing and stropping it. Such defects are quickly detected by the use of a microscope in the hands of an experienced and attentive observer.

The other method of testing the temper, while not infallible, will nevertheless be of assistance even to the most inexperienced. It consists of catching the point of the blade under the thumb nail, and then letting the nail slip off quickly. If the blade gives a good clear ring, you may conclude that it is well tempered, but if it does not ring full and clear it is an indication that the blade is tempered unevenly.

THE CONCAVE BLADE

The thinnest edge is always the sharpest. A blade ought therefore to be as thin as the strength of the metal composing it will permit. Nearly all razors are now made "hollow-ground" or "concave"—a great improvement over the old style of thick blade. The edge of the hollow-ground razor is thinner and therefore cuts better, and is much easier to keep sharp.

Almost any desired make of razor may be had in either half, three-quarters, or full concave. The full concave blade is of course the thinnest. In view of the fact that the thinner the edge the sharper the instrument, most purchasers of a razor quite naturally conclude that the full concave blade is the best. Our impression is that this is a mistake; that the full concave blade is not so good for shaving most beards as the three-quarters concave. In a very deeply hollow ground razor, the blade is ground extremely thin, back to a line some distance from the edge. When such an edge—almost as thin as paper—comes in contact with a stiff beard, unless the blade is held very flat upon the face, it is quite likely to bend and spring, and a cut will be the result.

WIDTH OF THE BLADE.

The width of the blade is another point that should receive attention. As a rule we believe the beginner selects too wide a blade. A comparatively narrow one, in the size known as the 4-8 is the best for most purposes, as it does not spring on the face so readily as the wide blade, yet it follows the contours of the face more closely, and in general is managed more easily.

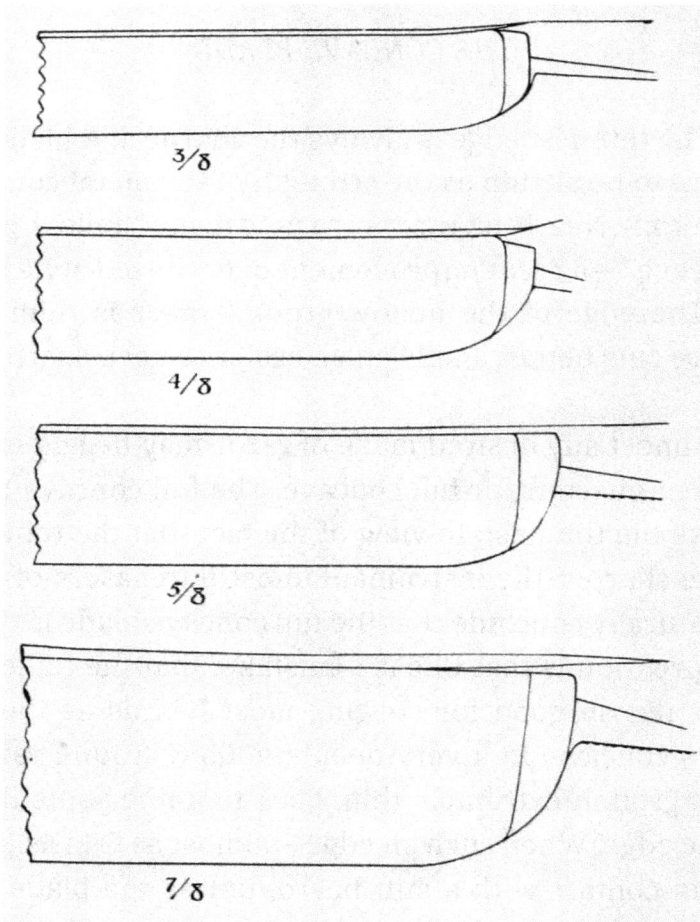

3/8

4/8

5/8

7/8

SHOWING DIFFERENT WIDTHS OF BLADES.

POINT OF THE BLADE.

The point of the razor ought to be slightly rounded as shown in the illustration. While this is seemingly a small matter, yet a sharp point has probably occasioned more cuts than almost any other cause. If you have a razor with a sharp point, you can round it off, on the edge of the hone. You should not use the top surface of the hone for this purpose, for if you do you are quite likely to scratch the hone and spoil it. Use water freely otherwise the blade will become heated and that would quickly spoil its temper.

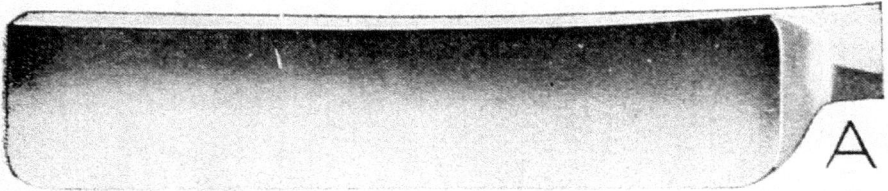

A.—THE ROUND POINTED BLADE.

B.—THE SHARP POINTED BLADE.

III.
CARE OF THE RAZOR.

Take good care of your razor. Many a fine razor has been spoiled by carelessness and neglect on the part of the user. The life of a razor will depend entirely on the care given it. Never put it away until it has first been wiped thoroughly dry, using a piece of chamois skin for this purpose. Even this will not remove all the moisture, so the blade should be drawn across the strop a few times, or else left exposed to the air for a few moments until the little particles of moisture not removed by the cloth have evaporated. Then you may replace the razor in its case with the expectation of finding it in good condition when you next use it.

Rusting must be prevented, especially upon the edge, which seems to rust more quickly than any other part of the blade. A tiny rust spot on this delicate line, by causing the metal to soften and crumble at that point, will soon end the usefulness of the razor, unless the edge is ground back past the rust spot. In such a case there is always the liability of not getting a good edge.

In wiping the lather off the blade never use a glazed or coarse paper. Tissue paper is the best. Many overlook this point and by drawing the blade straight across a glazed or hard finished paper, turn the edge, and then wonder why the razor has lost its keenness. Draw the blade over the paper obliquely, away from the edge, in the same direction as when stropping it.

IV.
THE SAFETY RAZOR.

Of recent years a great number of safety razors have been invented and placed on the market, the manufacturers of each claiming that theirs are superior to all others and that they have at last produced a razor that is destined to revolutionize shaving.

One thing may be said of safety razors in general—that if a man uses one he is less likely to cut himself, but this is all that can reasonably be said in their favor. Of course, if it were impossible to shave with the ordinary razor without cutting one's self, then the safety razor would become a necessity. The truth is, however, that anyone who has a good keen smooth-cutting razor, lathers the face thoroughly, and will learn—if he does not already know—how to handle the razor properly, will run almost no danger. Such a man will seldom cut himself.

On the other hand, most of the safety razors are difficult to keep clean and dry, and therefore free from rust; and owing to the difficulty of stropping them, it is almost, if not quite impossible to keep them sharp. It is also difficult to make the correct stroke with them. Probably a hundred thousand safety razors have been sold in the United States within the past few years and it is extremely doubtful if ten per cent. of them are now in use.

V.
THE HONE.

The edge of a razor, when viewed under a powerful microscope, presents an appearance very different from that seen by the unaided eye. Unmagnified, the edge appears to be a continuous unbroken line. Such actually is not the case, for the microscope reveals the fact that, instead of being straight and unbroken, the edge is in reality composed of a great number of minute points much resembling the teeth of a saw.

These points or teeth follow each other throughout the entire length of the blade, and by their extreme minuteness and unbroken regularity give the edge its exceeding keenness. Now if the razor becomes dull, these teeth will be less even and regular and their edges will be rounded and worn away. To sharpen the razor, therefore, it is necessary—by making the edge as thin as possible—to restore these little teeth to their original condition. This cannot be done by stropping, but is accomplished only by the process known as honing.

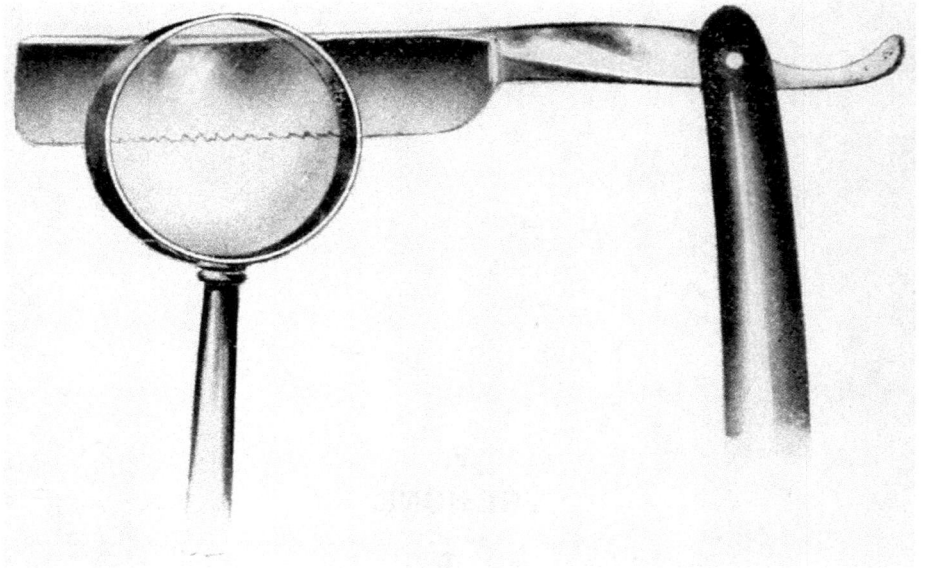

EDGE OF THE RAZOR AS IT APPEARS UNDER THE
MICROSCOPE.

It has been asserted by some, that when once the razor
has been ground and set, the strop alone without further honing
or grinding is sufficient to keep it in order. This opinion has
emanated from certain makers of razor-strops, who wish to
induce the public to purchase their goods. They represent their
strops as having been "metalized," or otherwise treated with
some kind of preparation that makes honing unnecessary. As a
rule, we would advise the reader to beware of these "wonder-
working-strops." Such preparations may, and sometimes do,
improve the strop, just as lather when applied to a strop will
improve it, but that they will do more than this, we deny.
When the special offices of the hone and of the strop are fully
understood, it will at once become apparent that no strop can
possibly take the place of a hone.

The object of honing a razor is to make its edge as *thin* and *flat* as a proper attention to the degree of firmness required will permit. This is accomplished by the hard fine grit of the hone cutting and wearing away the steel. The strop cannot do this. On the contrary, stropping a razor, instead of giving it a thin and flat edge, always has a tendency to produce a rounded one. This results from the very nature of the strop, which always "gives" or sags more or less during the process of stropping, and the more the strop is permitted to sag, the sooner will such an edge be produced, and in proportion as the edge assumes this rounded form, it losses its keenness. The flattest and thinnest edge is always the sharpest, and the only way to impart such an edge to a razor is by means of the hone.

Before explaining the process of honing, it may be well to say a word about the different kinds of hones, so that should the reader wish to purchase one, he may do it intelligently.

There are two distinct classes of hones in general use,— one known as the rock hone, on account of its being cut from the natural rock, and the other manufactured. A great number of hones are produced in different parts of the United States, but few that are really suitable for sharpening razors. A razor hone must be of the very finest quality. The natural stones are usually composed principally of silica, which is one of the sharpest cutting minerals known. It easily cuts the hardest steel and the fine grit imparts a very smooth edge to a razor. The "Arkansas," found near the famous Hot Springs, is one of this variety, but owing to the difficulty of obtaining this stone, and the great waste in cutting it, the supply is limited and the price high.

THE HONE.

Most of the razor hones used in the United States are imported. The most noted are the German water hones, the oil hones from Belgium, and the Swaty hones from Austria. The last named are very reasonable in price and quite a favorite among barbers. They are a manufactured hone, and in some respects the manufactured hones are superior to the natural stones, in that they are free from seams and uneven spots and perfectly uniform in texture.

Most men have the idea that honing is a difficult operation and should be undertaken only by expert cutlers or barbers. Very few seem to think that they can hone there own razors. How this impression became current, it is difficult to say. We venture to assert, however, that honing a razor is at least as easy as stropping it. In this case as in many others, the difficulty arises from supposing there is a difficulty.

How to Use the Hone

VI.
HOW TO USE THE HONE.

The hone being the only means of sharpening a dull razor, its use becomes at once of the utmost importance to those who wish to keep their razors in perfect order.

Hones are seldom used dry, but are usually covered with either water, lather or oil: first—to prevent heating the blade which would quickly spoil its temper; second—to keep the particles of steel that are ground off the blade from entering the pores of the stone, which would soon fill up and result in what is known as a glazed surface; and third—to make the surface of the hone as smooth as possible.

Before commencing the operation, wipe the hone clean, then put on a few drops of oil or else cover it with water or lather. This will float the little particles of steel ground off the razor, thus preventing them from remaining directly on the hone to impede its full and equal effect. With most hones you may use either water, lather or oil; but do not change from one to the other; whichever you begin with, use that exclusively. It requires a longer time to produce a keen edge when oil is used but the edge is somewhat smoother. Most barbers use lather and we should advise the beginner to do so.

Directions for Honing.

The hone, with its fine surface up, should be placed perfectly flat on a table or other solid foundation. (The rough surface is intended merely as a support and not for use.) After covering the hone with lather, place the razor flat upon it as shown in *Fig. A*. With the thumb and fore finger, grasp the razor back of the heel, so as to have firm hold of both the blade and the handle. Draw the blade from heel to point, forward against the edge, and with a moderate degree of pressure, until it comes into the position shown in *Fig. B*. Now, without lifting the blade from the stone, turn the edge up, so that the razor rests on the back of the blade. Slide it forward on its back from point to heel and let it fall into the position indicated in *Fig. C*. Push the blade from heel to point against the edge, finishing the stroke as in *Fig. D*. Turn the blade on its back, slide from point to heel and let it fall into the first position, as shown in *Fig. A*. Continue honing until the blade is sufficiently keen and free from nicks and inequalities. This may be known by drawing the edge, very lightly, across the moistened thumb nail. If it sticks to the nail slightly, it is an indication that the honing has developed the little teeth which constitute the perfect razor edge, and that the razor is now ready for stropping.

If the honing be carried too far, a "wire edge" will be produced, and this must be removed. To do this, draw the edge with a steady hand across the moistened thumb nail in the manner indicated above. The blade should then be drawn once or twice across the hone as before, in order to unite all parts of the edge and cause a perfect equality of keenness from

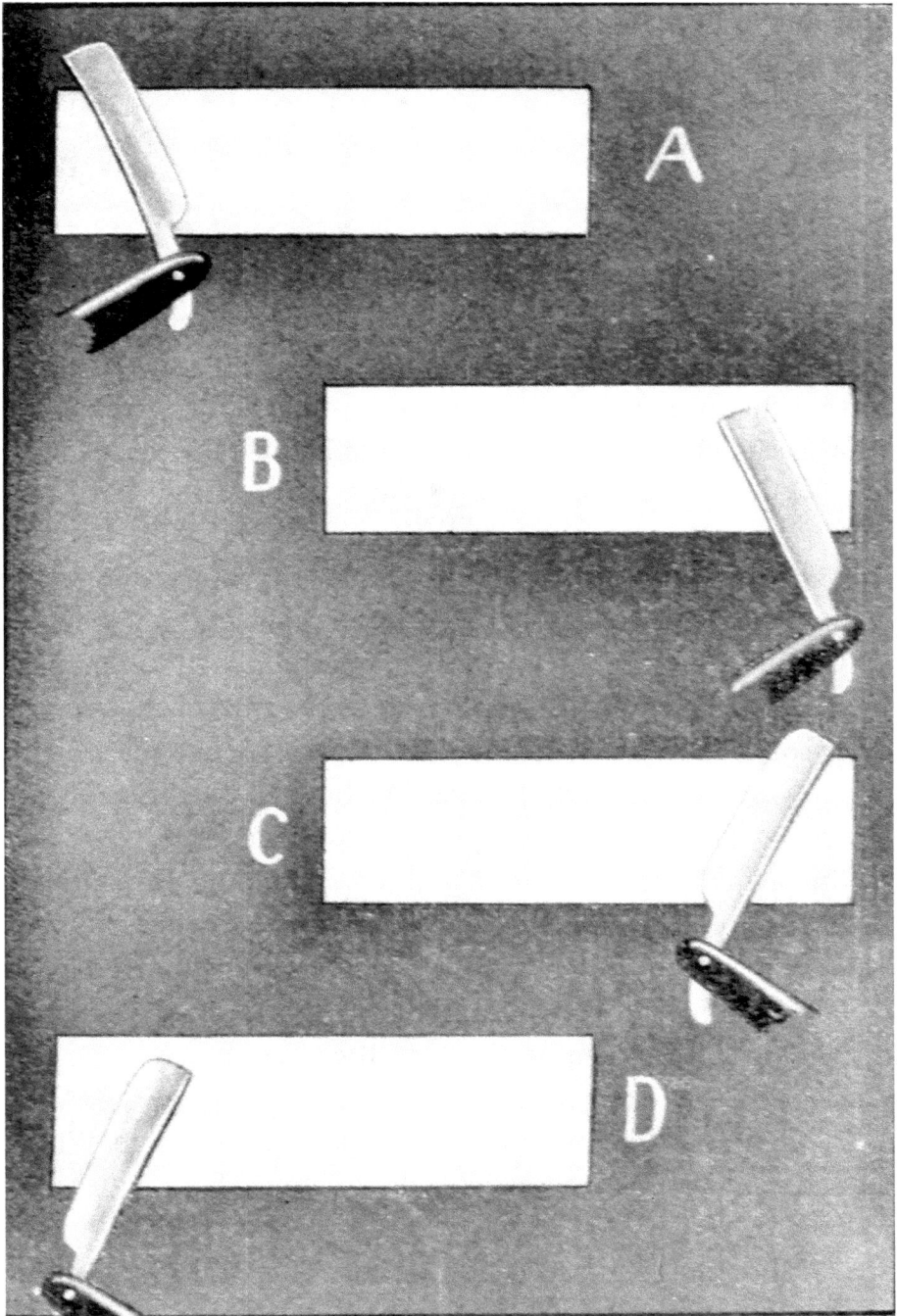

HOW TO HONE THE RAZOR

one end of the blade to the other. With this done, the operation is in general performed, and the wondrous difficulty of honing the razor vanishes.

Special Directions.

The following directions should be specially observed.

First—The blade should be held perfectly flat on the hone, so that the back, as well as the edge, touches the stone. If the back is raised from the stone so that only the edge touches, the bevel will be short and the edge blunt.

Second—In drawing the blade across the hone diagonally against the edge, the heel should be about one and a half inches in advance of the point, and care should be taken to maintain the same angle when the stroke is reversed and throughout the entire operation. This sets the teeth at the proper angle, that is, slightly inclined toward the heel. We have likened the edge of a razor to that of a saw, but there is this difference: saw teeth incline away from the handle and toward the point, while the razor teeth incline away from the point and toward the heel. This is correct in principle, for the saw in use is pushed away from the handle toward the point, while the razor is usually drawn away from the point toward the heel.

Third—Press with equal force on all parts of the edge. With a good hone, very little pressure will be required.

The time required to hone a razor depends much on the condition of the razor and the hardness of the steel composing it. When the edge is in the usual condition—that is when it is free from nicks and has merely become thick in consequence of the injudicious use of the razor strop—it will need very little honing; eight or ten strokes in each direction will be quite sufficient. When, however, the edge has nicks: though so small as to be scarcely perceptible, the operation will require more time and attention. Should the nicks be large, it will be better to send the razor to a cutler to be ground.

If the razor is well cared for and properly stropped, it will not require very frequent honing, probably not oftener than once in from six to eight weeks. When it is required you will become aware of it, from the fact that stropping will not sharpen it.

VII.
THE STROP.

The object of honing the razor, as has been explained, is to abrade and wear away the edge of the blade so that it becomes as thin as possible. But when this is done, the process of sharpening the razor is still incomplete, for the edge, when taken from the hone, is left rough and unfit to put on the face. Another process is necessary, and that is stropping. The object of stropping is not to make the blade thinner, but to smooth the edge, taking off the rough surface of the little teeth which have been developed, and setting them all in perfect alignment. This gives the razor its exceeding keenness.

You should have a first-class strop. It little matters how good your razor may be if your strop is a poor one, for it is absolutely impossible to keep a razor in good condition if the strop is of poor quality or rough and haggled. Many a razor has been blamed when the fault lie entirely with the strop and the manner of using it. So called sharpening preparations, sometimes applied to the surface of strops, as a substitute for the hone, should be avoided. Most of them contain acid or emery, which is likely to gradually spoil the temper of the razor.

There are many kinds of strops manufactured and placed on the market, some good and some bad. The most common is the swing strop, made of leather or horse hide on one side and canvas or hose on the other. Some of the cheaper grades have a very coarse canvas, and unless you wish to ruin your razor, you should never put it on such a strop. In our opinion a good leather or horse hide strop is the best, and meets every requirement; but if a combination strop is used, the linen or hose side should be of the finest quality.

The strop should be not less than twenty inches long and two inches wide. Its surface should be very soft and smooth—not glazed—and you can tell whether it is so, by rubbing the hand over it. Do not fold the strop when putting it away, for if you do you are likely to crack or roughen the surface, and this will injure the edge of the blade when it is drawn across it.

Care of the Strop.

After the strop has been put to a great deal of use, it will sometimes be found that it will not "take hold" on the razor—that is it will allow the blade to slip over it with little or no resistance and thus fail to impart a keen, smooth-cutting edge. The reason is that the strop has become dry and porous. Do not attempt to remedy the matter by applying oil or razor paste; these will only make matters worse. Hang the strop on a hook, and with the left hand stretch as tightly as possible. Apply a good thick lather to the surface and rub it in with the palm of the hand. Barbers sometimes nail the strop to a board and rub the lather in with a smooth bottle; but the hand will do quite as well, and indeed, we think it preferable. What the strop requires is to have the pores filled with the lather; so put on and work in coat after coat, until the leather will take up no more. Then leave the strop to dry. This simple treatment will completely change the action of the strop, and the next time you use it, you will be surprised and delighted to note its improved effect on the razor. It will have that "cling" and "resistance" which barbers so much desire in a strop, and which, indeed, is quite essential to its efficiency.

VIII.
HOW TO STROP THE RAZOR.

Place a hook in a door or a window casing about four or five feet from the floor. Put the ring of the strop over the hook, and hold the handle firmly in the left hand as shown in the accompanying illustration. The strop should be pulled tight—not allowed to hang loosely—otherwise the edge of the razor will become rounded and require frequent honing.

Open the razor, so that the handle is in line with the blade. Grasp it firmly with the right hand, the first two fingers and thumb holding the razor just back of the heel, so that perfect control is had of both the blade and handle. With the razor held in this manner it is an easy matter to turn the razor back and forth from one side to the other.

Lay the blade flat on the further end of the strop, as shown in Fig. E, with the edge away from you. Draw the blade toward you, always keeping the heel of the razor in advance of the point. When at the end of the strop, rotate the razor on its back till the unstropped side of the blade comes in contact with the strop, as shown in Fig. F. Then, with the heel in advance, push the razor away from you, until it reaches the further end of the strop. Again rotate, and continue the stropping until the razor is sharp.

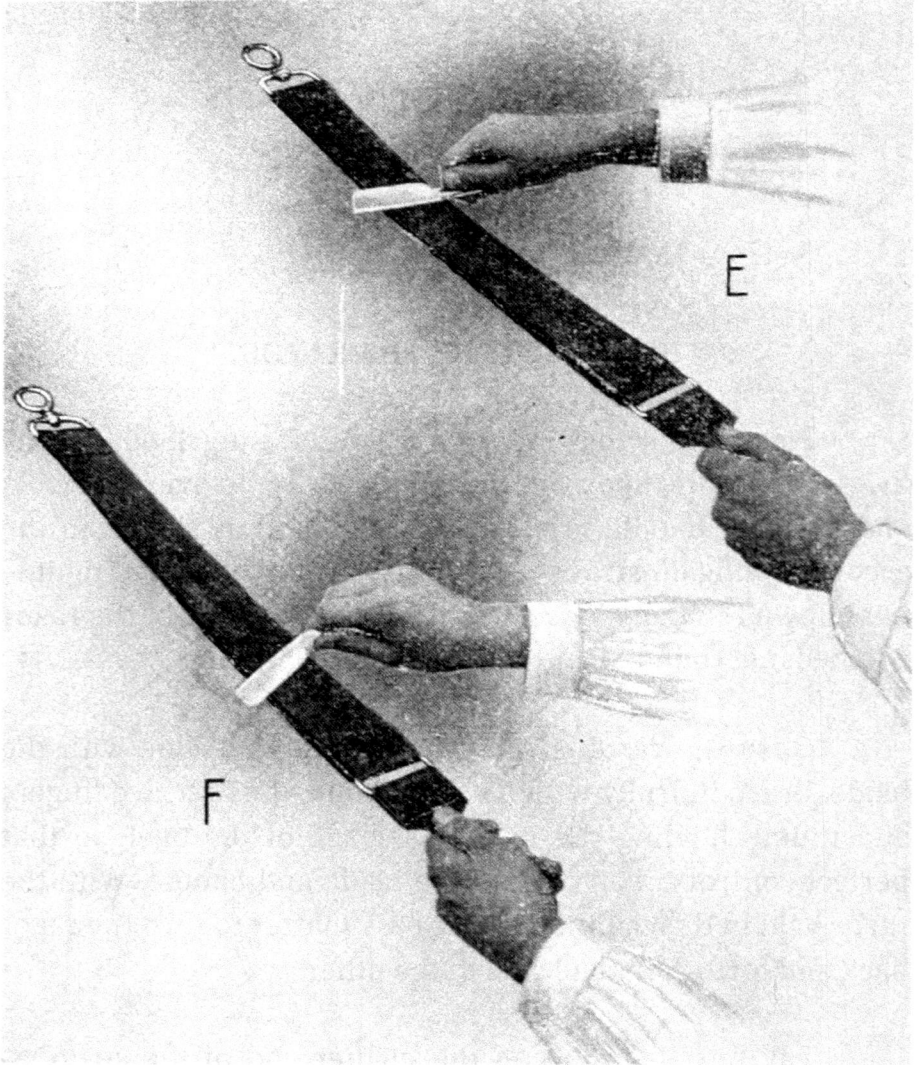

HOW TO STROP THE RAZOR.

Always hold the blade at the same angle, and perfectly flat on the strop. You will observe that the stroke is exactly opposite to that used in honing. In honing, the edge is in advance; in stropping, the back. During the operation the back of the razor should never be taken from the strop. By observing this, and always turning the blade on its back, instead of on the edge, you will avoid cutting the strop.

Beginners should not attempt to make a quick stroke. Let the stroke be slow and even, developing speed gradually until a complete mastery of the movement is acquired.

If the razor is in good condition and not in need of honing, fifteen or twenty strokes in each direction will be sufficient. If, however, the razor should require honing, no amount of stropping will put a keen edge on it. It will usually be necessary to strop the razor each time you shave, and with stiff beards more than once may be required.

IX.
THE BRUSH.

Purchase a good brush. The cheap ones are usually the most expensive in the end, and nearly always prove unsatisfactory. It should be remembered that the vital part of a brush is in the setting, and particular attention should therefore be paid to that part of it. Cheap brushes are commonly set with glue, rosin or cement, which soon cracks and becomes unadhesive; whereupon the bristles fall out. We recommend a brush made of bristles or badger hair and set in hard vulcanized rubber. A brush so constructed, with wood, bone or ivory handle, and hard rubber ferule, will not shed the bristles or crack open, and with proper care will last for years.

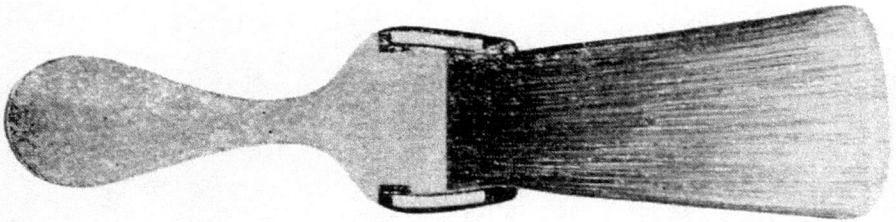

SECTIONAL VIEW OF THE BRUSH SHOWING INTERNAL CONSTRUCTION.

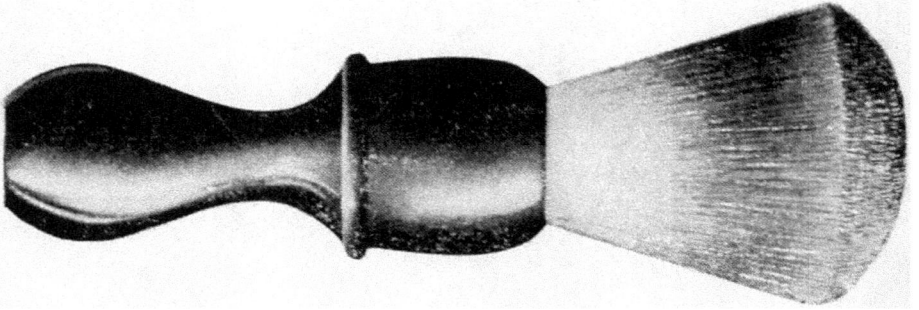

THE BRUSH.

Do not leave the lather to dry in the brush, but after shaving rinse it out thoroughly and dry the brush with a towel, before putting away. The cup and brush should be kept clean and away from dust. Once a week they should be washed with hot water.

X.
THE CUP.

The shaving cup should be of earthen ware or china, and large enough to accommodate the ordinary round cake of shaving soap. Some cups are made with two compartments, one for soap and the other for water, but this arrangement is unnecessary, and in fact, not so convenient as the ordinary cup, for it leaves too little room for making the lather.

If possible, the cake of soap should entirely fill the bottom of the cup so that no space is left between the soap and the sides: otherwise water will get in and keep the bottom of the cake[Pg 49] continually soaked. If it is found that the cake does not quite fill the space, take the soap out and warm it until it becomes somewhat soft, then put it back in the cup, and with the hand press down the sides all around, thus flattening out the cake until it quite fills the intervening space. If at any time the soap should cleave away from the sides of the cup, it should be pressed back as at first. This will be found the most convenient way of using the soap.

Great care should be taken to keep the cup scrupulously clean, rinsing it out thoroughly each time after shaving, in order to remove any lather that may have been left unused. Keep the cup away from dust.

Some use the sticks of shaving soap and make the lather on the face. While this is permissible, we think the better way is to make the lather in the cup and put it on with the brush.

XI.
THE SOAP.

Next to the razor, the most important article of the shaving outfit is the soap. In its proper use lies the real secret of easy shaving. The razor may be ever so good, but unless the beard is properly lathered with a good soap, shaving will be anything but a pleasure. Use only a regular recognized standard make of shaving soap, not, under any circumstances, a toilet soap. The latter is not intended for shaving, and is likely to produce irritations of the skin and leave the face rough and sore.

A wrong idea prevails regarding the use of the soap. The popular impression is that the soap is used for the purpose of softening the beard, in which condition it is supposed to be most easily cut. This is a mistake. The soap is used, not to soften the beard, but to produce exactly the opposite effect—namely, to make the hair stiff and brittle, so that they will present a firm and resisting surface to the razor. A hair, as is well known, is a tube composed of a hard fibrous substance, growing from a bulb or root, which secretes an oily matter. This oil works its way up through the hair, and by permeating all parts, renders the hair soft and pliable. Now in this natural oily condition, it is very difficult to cut the hair with a razor, and it becomes even more difficult if the beard be made still softer by the application of hot water. Many do this, and it is no wonder they find shaving difficult. When this is done, the hairs become soft and limp, and the razor will either slip over them entirely, or else cut partly into them, bend them back and slice them lengthwise, all the while pulling and straining them at the roots, and making the process of shaving most painful. Now soap has the opposite effect. It contains either alkali, potash or soda, which when applied to the beard in the form of lather, unites with the oil of the hair, neutralizing it and removing it, and renders the hairs hard stiff and brittle—in which condition they may be easily and readily cut. For the sake of cleanliness, the face should, of course, be washed previous to shaving in order to remove any dirt or grit from the beard, which might dull the razor; but before applying the lather, the face should be well dried with a towel.

XII.
THE LATHER.

To make the lather, see that the soap is placed in the cup according to previous directions. Fill the cup with water, allowing it to stand for a few seconds, then pour the water out. Usually sufficient water to make the lather will adhere to the cup, soap and brush. Now with the brush, mix thoroughly, using a combined stirring and churning motion, until a good thick lather appears. The more the brush is rubbed over the soap the thicker the lather becomes. A great deal depends upon having the lather just right. If it is thin and watery, you will have poor success in shaving. The more creamy it is, the better will be the effect of the alkali in stiffening the beard. Some of the poorer qualities of soap produce lather very quickly, sometimes half filling the cup, but it will be found thin and without lasting qualities, so that by the time one side of the face has been shaved, the lather is all gone from the other. A good soap will produce a thick creamy lather that will last throughout the entire process of shaving.

Applying the Lather.

Put the lather on with the brush, covering every part of the face that you intend to shave. Then with the fingers rub it thoroughly into the beard until the lather has had sufficient time to stiffen the hairs. Next to having the razor in perfect condition, this is the most important thing to do; for it is impossible to shave easily unless the face is well lathered and the lather thoroughly worked into the beard. Go over the face once more with the brush, in order to spread the lather evenly, and then begin shaving at once, before the lather has time to dry. Should it dry while you are shaving, wet the brush slightly and apply fresh lather. If you prepare your face in accordance with these instructions, a keen razor will slip over the face so easily that shaving will become a real pleasure.

XIII.
INSTRUCTIONS TO BEGINNERS.

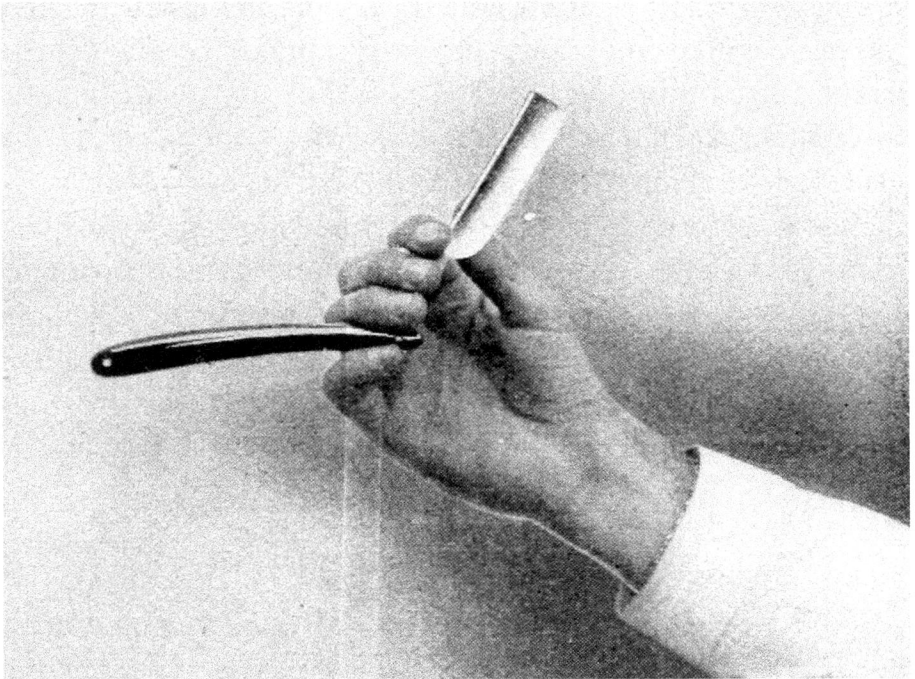

THE RIGHT WAY TO HOLD THE RAZOR

If you are a young man, just beginning to shave, it is important that you commence right. It is quite as easy to learn the right way as the wrong way. Do not entertain the idea that it is a difficult matter for one to shave himself—for there is nothing difficult about it when you know how. You may have previously tried and failed, but if you will now follow the instructions contained in this book, there is no reason why shaving may not be performed without further difficulties.

The accompanying illustration shows the position in which the razor should be held. It will be observed that the handle is thrown well back past the heel. The first three fingers rest on the back of the blade, with the little finger over the crook at the end, and the thumb on the side of the blade, near the middle. In this position, with the handle acting as a balance, the razor will be under perfect control, and there will be little danger of cutting oneself. This position can be maintained throughout most of the process of shaving, although it may be necessary to change it slightly while shaving certain parts, as for instance the neck, under the jaw. But whatever the position, endeavor to have the razor at all times under perfect control. The position here indicated, is the one we should certainly advise the beginner to adopt, but if a man, from long continued use has formed the habit of holding the razor in a different way, any change will prove difficult and may not be advisable.

The Stroke.

Owing no doubt largely to individual temperament, there is considerable variation in the manner of using the razor, with different persons. Some find a long slow stroke best, while others make it short and quick. Each man must suit the stroke to his own convenience. But certain principles are applicable to everybody. In the first place you should begin with a slow even stroke, gradually increasing it as you gain better control of the razor. Speed will develop naturally with practice.

Hold the razor quite flat upon the face. Do not pull the razor directly down against the beard, but hold it obliquely to the direction of movement. In general shave in the direction of the growth of the beard, like this:

Shaving against the growth pulls the hairs and thus

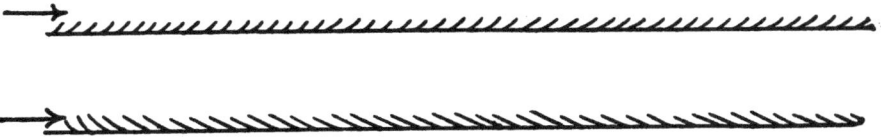

irritates the skin, and if the beard is heavy and wiry the edge of the blade is quite liable to catch in the hairs and be deflected inward and cut the face.

Position of the Mirror.

The mirror should hang between two windows if possible, so that when you look into it the light will fall directly upon both sides of your face. You will then be able to get a good reflection of either side. Remove the collar. To prevent soiling the shirt, place a towel around the neck in an easy, comfortable manner, pinning it at the side.

The Right Way to Shave.

XIV.
THE RIGHT WAY TO SHAVE.

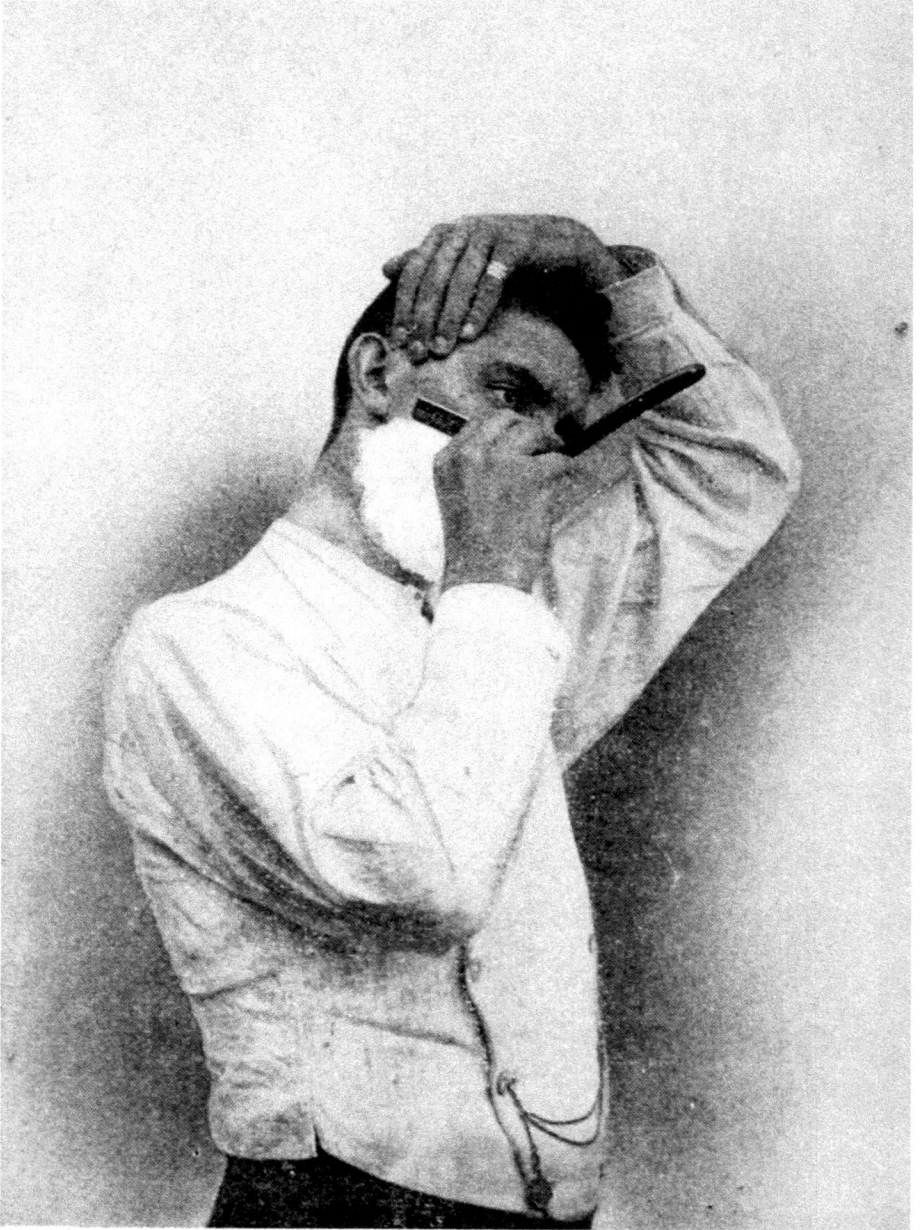

TO SHAVE THE RIGHT SIDE OF THE FACE.

TO SHAVE THE RIGHT SIDE OF THE FACE.

Reach over the head with the left hand and with the fingers draw the skin upward, thus making a smooth shaving surface. The illustration shows the proper position. Shave downward until about half of the right cheek is shaved, then slide the left hand still further over until the fingers rest in the middle of the cheek and again pull the skin upward. Now continue to shave downward until the entire right side of the face is shaved clean, as far as the middle of the chin and well under the jaw.

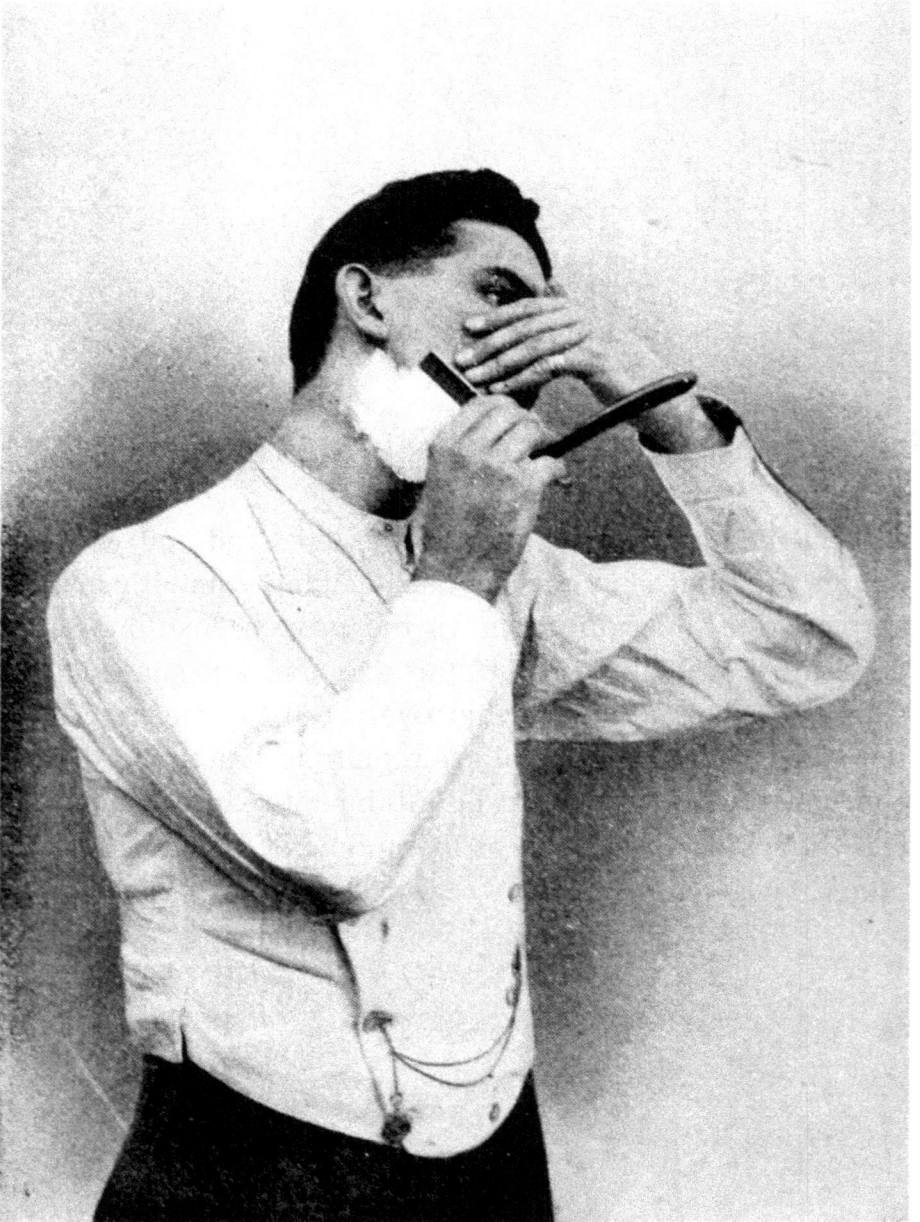

TO SHAVE THE RIGHT SIDE OF THE FACE UNDER THE JAW.

TO SHAVE THE RIGHT SIDE OF THE FACE UNDER THE JAW.

Hold the head over toward the left side with the chin slightly elevated. With the fingers of the left hand, draw the skin tight under the jaw. Shave downward if the beard grows in that direction; if not reverse the stroke. You should never shave against the growth when going over the face the first time, if it can be avoided. Keep the skin as tightly drawn as possible, for a better shaving surface is thus presented to the razor, and there is less liability of cutting yourself.

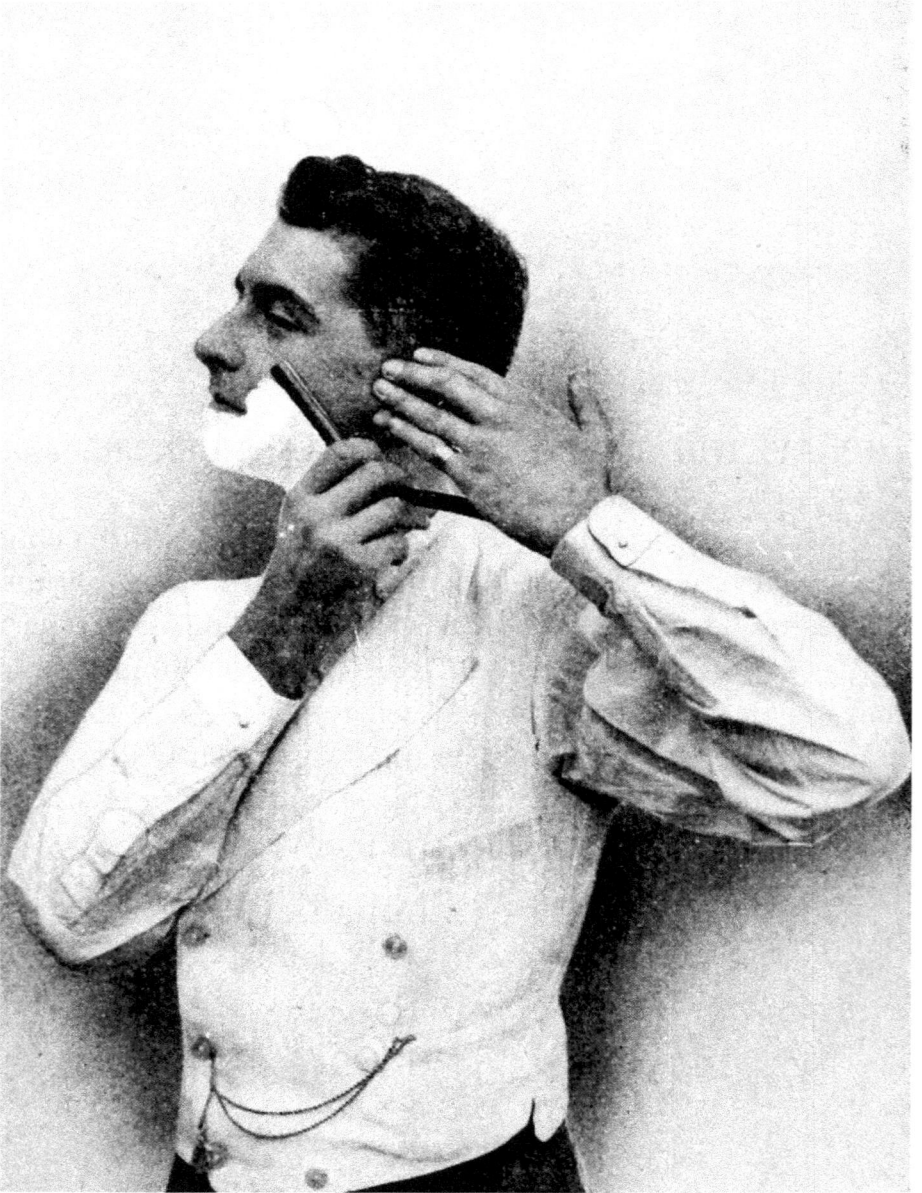

TO SHAVE THE LEFT SIDE OF THE FACE.

TO SHAVE THE LEFT SIDE OF THE FACE.

Place the fingers of the left hand in front of and just above the ear and press upward so as to draw the skin smooth on the upper left cheek. With the razor in the right hand, toe pointing upward, reach across the face as shown above, and shave downward. In shaving the lower part of the cheek and chin, follow downward with the left hand, keeping the skin tightly drawn.

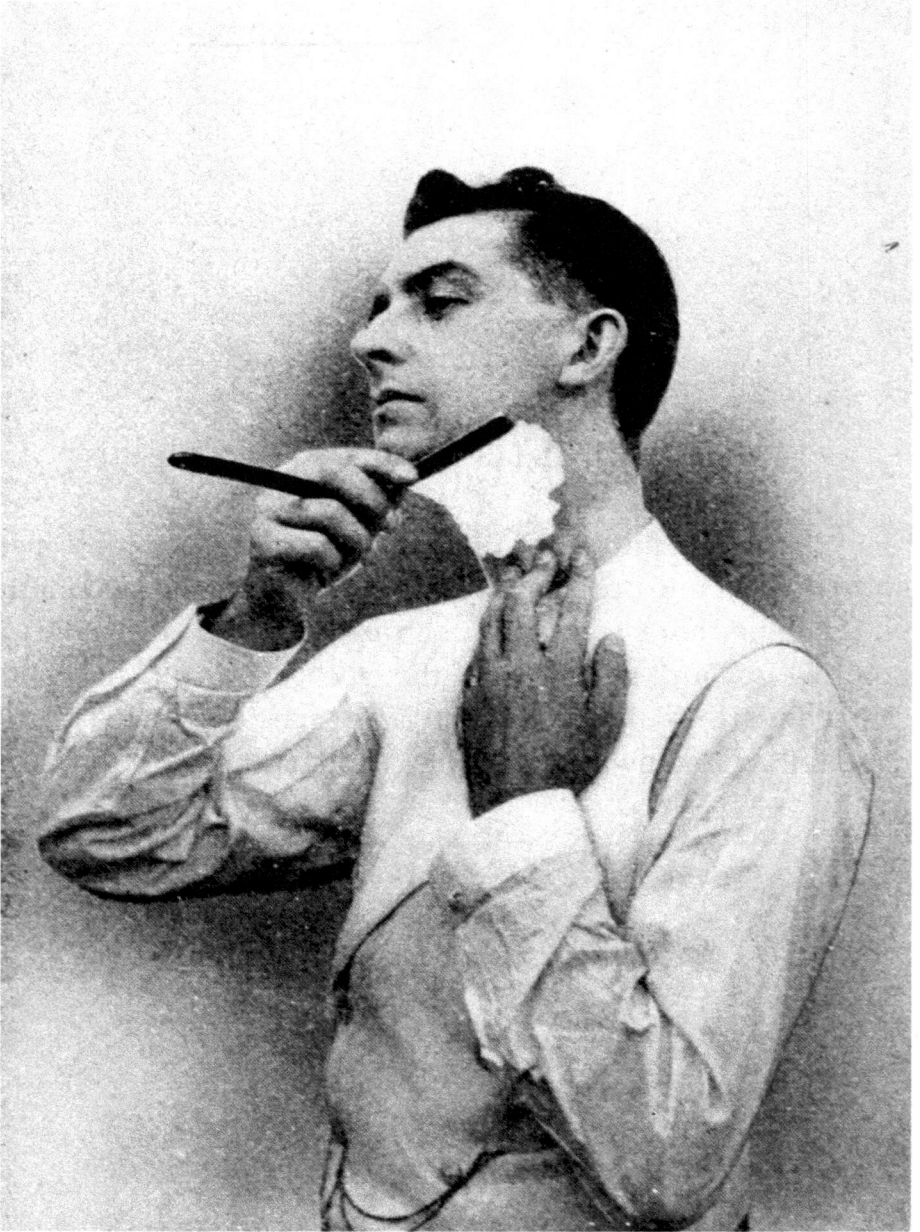

TO SHAVE THE LEFT SIDE OF THE FACE UNDER THE JAW.

TO SHAVE THE LEFT SIDE OF THE FACE UNDER THE JAW.

For many, this is the most difficult part of the face to shave as the skin is very tender, and unless treated gently will soon become irritated and sore. To shave easily, raise the chin, incline the head toward the right, and draw the skin as tight as possible with the left hand. Shave downward unless, as sometimes happens, the beard grows in the opposite direction, in which case you will, of course, reverse the stroke.

To shave the upper lip, draw the lip down as much as possible, to tighten the skin. Owing to the strong muscle in the lip, you will hardly need to use the left hand for this purpose.

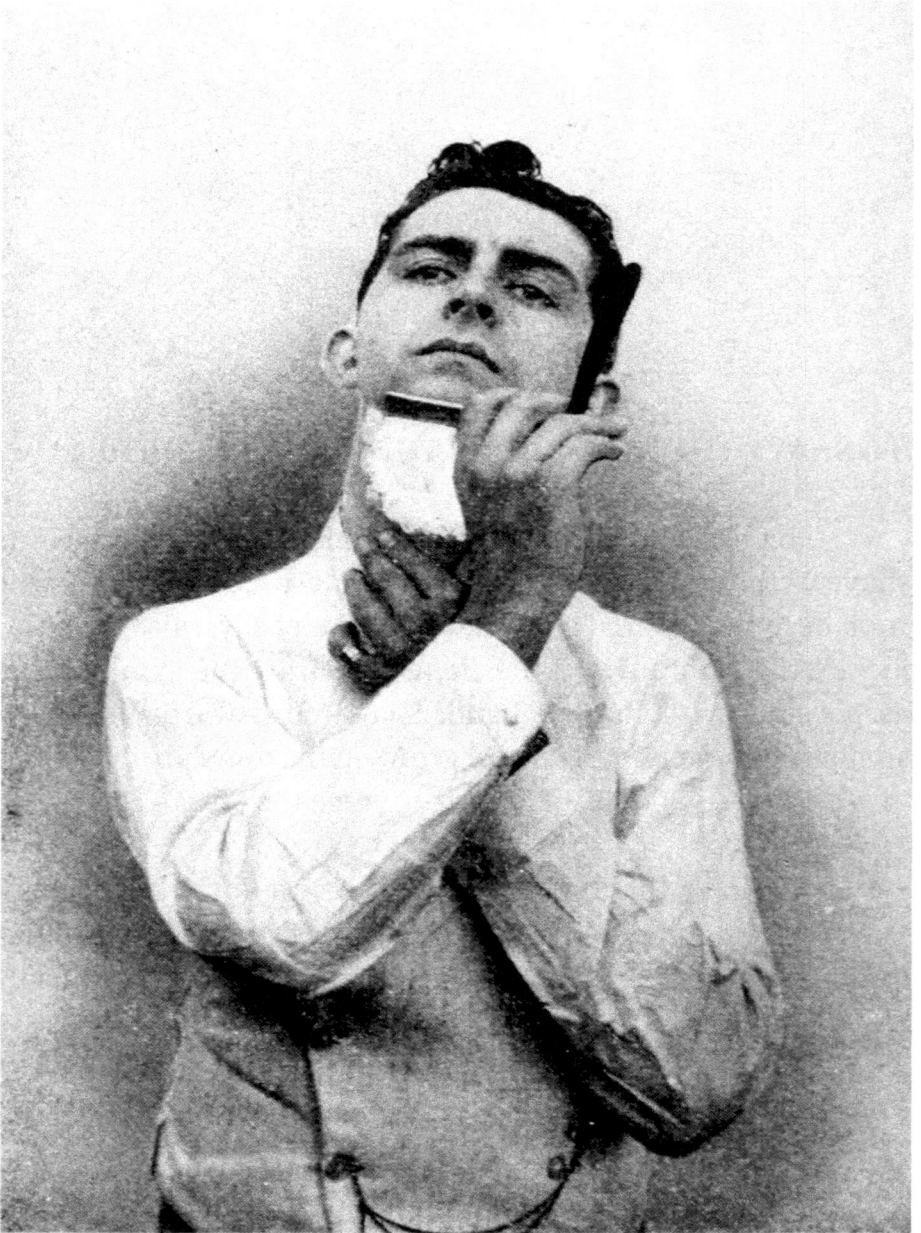

TO SHAVE UNDER THE CHIN.

TO SHAVE UNDER THE CHIN.

Throw the head backward and elevate the chin. Hold the razor in the right hand, and with the fingers of the left hand draw the skin downward. You should always endeavor to keep the skin drawn as smooth as possible, for by so doing you will greatly lessen the liability of cutting yourself and will be able to shave much more easily.

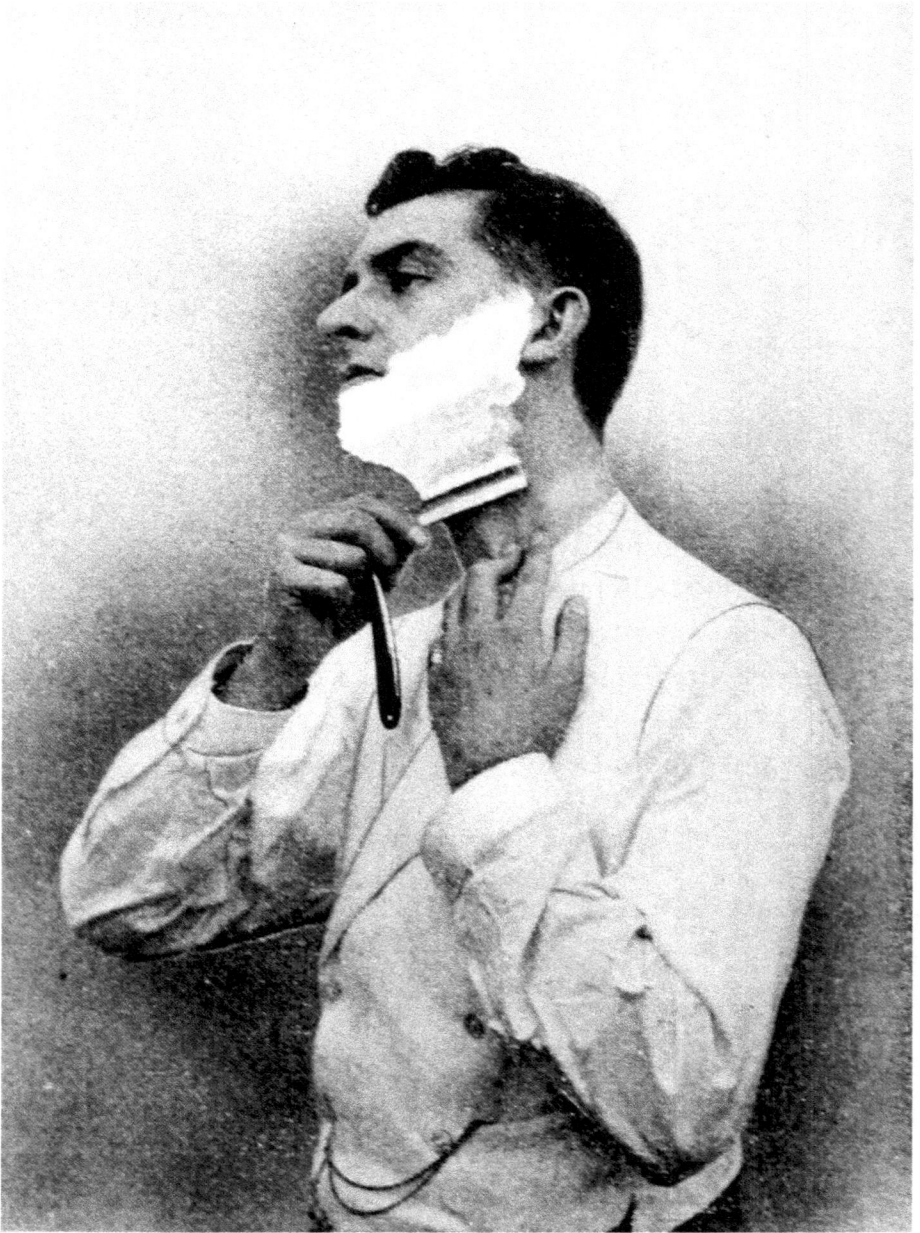

TO SHAVE UPWARD AGAINST THE GROWTH OF THE BEARD.

SHAVING OVER THE SECOND TIME.

If you desire a really clean shave, you must go over the face the second time. Strop the razor a few times before beginning. Lather the face as before, though it is unnecessary to rub the lather in with the fingers. Simply put it on with the brush.

In shaving over the face the second time, some reverse the stroke. That is, they shave upward against the growth of the beard, instead of downward, as during the first time over. This gives an exceedingly close shave and if the beard is stiff and heavy and the skin thin and tender, it may make the face sore, and cause the hairs to grow inward, under the skin. Perhaps the best way will be to shave lightly over the face the second time, in the same direction as at first. Each man should decide this point according to his own experience.

XV.
CARE OF THE FACE AFTER SHAVING.

Most men who shave themselves seem to think that when they have removed the beard, they have nothing further to do. This is a great mistake. They undervalue the importance of a proper treatment of the face. A quick and easy way of caring for the face after shaving, is to remove the lather by a thorough washing, then to apply either witch hazel, bay rum or some other good face lotion, and to follow this with a small quantity of talcum powder, evenly applied. This is probably about all that the average man will usually find time to do.

In order to keep the skin in a healthful condition, a little more elaborate treatment should occasionally be given. We recommend the following: Wash the face thoroughly to free it from the lather, and then apply a steaming hot towel, as hot as can be borne. The heat and moisture draw the blood to the face, open the pores, and set up a healthful action of the skin. Next apply witch hazel, and finally give the face a thorough massage. There is no other treatment so beneficial to the skin. With many persons the flow of blood to the face and scalp is very sluggish, because of enfeebled or slow heart action; and in consequence, the many small arteries and capillaries become clogged. Massage stimulates the circulation, and brings the blood from the inner centers to the surface, filling the many minute capillaries just underneath the skin, thus producing a tonic effect, which gives the skin renewed vigor and health.

What to do for a Cut.

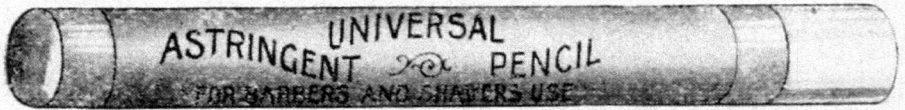

If a man cuts himself while shaving, it is usually due to certain causes that are easily avoidable. The principal causes are six in number:

First—Attempting to shave with a dull razor.

Second—Using a sharp pointed razor.

Third—Shaving with a razor that is too hollow ground, so that the edge springs and bends on the face.

Fourth—Holding the razor improperly.

Fifth—Shaving upward against the growth of the beard.

Sixth—Shaving in too great a hurry.

If you will avoid these mistakes and exercise proper care, you will seldom cut yourself. But when you do, it will be well to know how to treat the wound. If it be slight, the bleeding may sometimes be checked by using pressure. Covering the fingers with a towel, simply press the cut together. If this does not stop the flow, use an astringent. The styptic pencils, made especially for this purpose, are the best, and may be obtained at any store where barbers' supplies are kept. In case you should not have the pencils, alum may be used. In any event do not be discouraged, for such accidents sometimes happen to the best barbers.

XVI.
IRRITATION OF THE SKIN—ITS CAUSE AND PREVENTION.

Some men almost always experience burning and irritation of the skin after shaving. To such, we wish to offer some suggestions, which we hope will greatly benefit, if not entirely prevent the trouble.

The most common cause of irritation is undoubtedly a dull razor. If the razor is keen and sharp, the hairs will yield readily to the blade and no irritation will be produced. But if the blade is dull, instead of cutting the hairs easily, it passes over some, slices other lengthwise, and pulls and strains at the roots of all. This necessitates scraping the face over and over again, in order to get a clean shave, and the result is an irritation that perhaps continues until you are ready to shave again. Thus the tender parts of the skin are kept in a state of continual irritation. The remedy is of course, to see that the razor is always keen and sharp.

Another cause that may be mentioned, is chafing of the neck by the collar. If the edge of the collar is worn and rough, and comes in contact with the tender skin, it is sure to make it sore.

Too close shaving is a frequent cause, and those who are troubled in this way will do well to shave over the face but once.

Some of the cheap toilet waters are adulterated, and contain ingredients which undoubtedly produce a bad effect on the skin. In using bay rum or other face lotions, use only the best. If much trouble is experienced, we should advise the use of pure distilled witch hazel, which may be obtained at any drug store. This is soothing to the face and allays the burning.

Sometimes the trouble is due to an excess of alkali or potash in the soap. The best shaving soaps are especially prepared and have antiseptic and demulcent properties, which render them practically non-irritating. After shaving, take care to remove all the soap from the face; for during the process, the lather has been worked into the pores of the skin, and only by means of a thorough washing can it all be removed.

Irritations resulting from constitutional disease, or impurity of the blood, should, of course, be treated by a physician.

Some men are more subject to irritation of the skin than others. Those who have a thin and tender skin and a heavy and stiff beard, are especially liable, but with care, even these may prevent most of the trouble.